Ventilator

A COVID-19 Survivor Story

By: Deion Campbell

(Ventilator – A COVID-19 Survivor Story)
Copyright © 2020 by (Written By: Deion Campbell)

All rights reserved. No part of this book may be reproduced or transmitted in any form or by any means without written permission from the author.

ISBN#: 9798552249176
Printed in USA by Amazon (www.amazon.com)

Dedication

This book is my experience with the global coronavirus pandemic. Everything in this book is true, and has changed my life forever. I wrote this book to educate people who may currently have Covid-19, or somehow believe that it is not real and can't happen to them. This is for all those who believe wearing a mask, does not make a difference. Hopefully by sharing my pain, someone will wake up and realize that this pandemic is real. I do not encourage living in fear. I only want people to be aware of what's going on, and do their best to protect each other while making the world a better place. At the time of me writing this book, there is currently no vaccine for the virus available to the public. There have been at least 8 million cases reported, and over 200,000 Covid-19 related deaths in the United States of America. The United States is projected to reach a total of 400,000 deaths by January 2021.

If you have any questions, or would like to contact me; you can reach me by email or on social media.

ALL Social Media: *@Kinglegend757*
Email: Kinglegend757@gmail.com

Table of Contents

Dedication 3
Chapter 1 – Living My Best Life 5
Chapter 2 – Life or Death 13
Chapter 3 – Dream or Reality 22
Chapter 4 – Deja Vu.. 34
Chapter 5 – Road to Recovery....................... 42
Chapter 6 – Rehab.. 51
Chapter 7 – Home Sweet Home 59
Chapter 8 – Depression 65
Chapter 9 – Roadblocks 71
Chapter 10 – Reflection 79
Chapter 11 – What Now? 84
Chapter 12 – Intervention 90
Frequently Asked Questions – 96

Chapter One: Living my Best Life

Dear reader, I decided to write this book as a letter written just for you. Imagine opening my story from an envelope, while you sitting on the couch sipping on your favorite cup of wine or coffee. By the time you complete reading this letter, hopefully, we will have a cure to the coronavirus that took the world by storm.

Honestly, I don't believe anybody saw this global pandemic coming, at the very least the general public in the United States of America. Before I tell you about my experience with Covid-19, I'd like to share with you a little about myself and exactly who I am. Well to starts things off properly, my name is Deion Campbell and I was an upcoming photographer/videographer working on my brand, "King Legend 757."

I am currently married to a lovely wife, and we have a little Yorkie named Ricco Bentley Campbell. My wife and I loved to travel and take as many flights and road trips as possible. We met back in Elementary School; we both were born and raised in Hampton, Virginia we also graduated from Phoebus High School. No, we did not date while were in school, but we became friends and knew of each other's family because we were also neighbors who lived on the same street.

So you can basically say I have known my wife my entire life. One thing my wife could tell you about me is that I am very ambitious and have always wanted to be an Entrepreneur. As a photographer/videographer, I enjoyed capturing moments of a lifetime with my camera and was always eager to connect with new people by networking/collaborating on projects.

My passion in life was photography because I enjoyed giving people a reason to smile and being involved with people who trusted me with their most precious moments in life. Weddings, Birthdays, Events, and more, I was there to capture it all. I even ended up on a billboard in my city on interstate 64 and captured my first concert at the Hampton Coliseum.

I remember receiving a video shout-out from Actor, Tiny Lister who is also known as "Debo," from his famous role in the hit movie "Friday." Once the video was posted on Instagram it received over 1 MILLION VIEWS, after the shade room reposted it. From that point on, I ended up being well known in the area and eventually would be contacted for interviews on radio stations, online blogs, and media outlets.

I have always been a firm believer in creating opportunities and not waiting for them to come to me. Sometimes in life, you won't see a change until you become the change. From the moment I picked up a camera, I was determined to be the very best and make a name for myself.

I remember starting my Instagram and going to events where nobody knew who I was. My first 1,000 followers came from giving away free photos taken at events in exchange for a follow on Instagram. I was doing everything for free. I was growing my brand fast, and gaining that exposure at the same time.

Things for my brand really took flight when I ended up networking with local DJ J Skillz. Every venue he would DJ at, I ended up snapping photos as his personal photographer. Eventually, people got used to seeing my face, and I became established locally in my area.

From Virginia, I took my camera with me everywhere I went, back and forth trips to Philadelphia, Las Vegas, Miami, Key West, Bahamas, Cozumel Mexico, North Carolina, Washington D.C., and to my final trip to Atlanta during the beginning of the COVID 19 era in the United States of America.

The month was February 2020 when my wife and I took our flight to visit Atlanta for the first time. I remember enjoying the city very much. We visited the Coca-Cola factory, checked in at Celebrity photographer Cam Kirk Studios, went to Lenox Mall, got drinks and relaxed at the Sky Lounge, and enjoyed a full-access VIP tour of CNN.

I remember walking inside of CNN and learning so much about the world news broadcasting system, and how it works. I saw the behind the scenes of what goes on behind the stories we see on television. At the time I visited, Kobe Bryant's tragic death from the helicopter crash in Calabasas, California was the most trending topic.

One of the things I remember the most about staying in downtown Atlanta was the lack of drive-through fast-food restaurants. You have to pay for parking everywhere and there is almost nowhere to park close to the building you need to get to.

I know that sounds normal to city life, but in my city where I am from, we have parking spaces in front of businesses that don't require a parking meter or garage. We have parking spaces available everywhere. I guess that's the humor in the saying, "there is no place like home".

One of the things that caught my attention the most about Atlanta was how diverse the population was. Seeing Caucasian people hang out with African American people was not a normal picture for me. They blended in a way that seemed unbelievable to me. In Hampton, VA there isn't much diversity. It's either black or white. We have a very few Asian/Latino population here.

Whether it is on purpose or a subconscious decision, blacks tend to hang with blacks and whites tend to hang with whites. That's the picture I have always had to look at since I was born in the year of 1993. I can't speak for the entire city of Atlanta, but from what I saw when I visited for that short period, was something that Martin Luther King definitely dreamed about.

After my wife and I returned home to Virginia from our weekend trip to Atlanta, I remember hitting another milestone in my life. Actually capturing photos at the BIGGEST event venue in the entire Hampton Roads area. To me, this was reaching another level of being a photographer/videographer.

This was my first opportunity to shine and really make a name for myself in the industry. I was placed in a position to capture my first concert. Jam Jam 2020, included big-name celebrities such as hip-hop artist, Da Baby, Pop Smoke, Gunna, and Stunna 4 Vegas. All put together by Big-Will Tha Party King.

There were so many people in attendance, and I was in the front row, moving in and out through to crowd to capture different angles. I also had access to backstage. I literally took thousands of photos that night, and also recorded a highlight video of the event.

This was the moment in my career where I can honestly say, I felt like all my hard work had actually paid off. I had truly started to feel myself; it was kind of hard not too. I had just received a video shout out from celebrity actor Tiny Lister telling people to book me, which hit over 1 MILLION views on Instagram.

I traveled to one of the biggest Celebrity Photographer Studios in the Country. I was getting interviewed on radio shows, online blogs, and media outlets. I had a VIP tour of the biggest news company in the world at CNN.

I flew back home to see myself on a larger than life billboard on interstate 64 and was now shooting my first concert at one of the biggest, well-respected venues in the entire state of Virginia. That's a whole lot of milestones to process at one time.

Now that I can look back on it, I became too big for myself. I had truly became "King Legend" and started to lose who Deion Campbell was. One thing that I would soon learn about life is that it will always find a way to remind you of your roots or where you came from.

We spend our entire lives chasing a dream that was born in the mind of a person who was still not fully aware of what is best for their own future. Life is all about trial and error, learning from life experiences, and maturing as an adult.

The moment you think you learned a lesson, life hits you with a more challenging one. This cycle continues over and over again until we leave this Earth. I believe the ultimate goal in life is to inspire and motivate others to follow their dreams.

That way when they accomplish it, they can inspire another to do the same. As Denzel Washington would say, "Each one, Teach one." My biggest life lesson was yet to come, but lord knows it was on its way faster than a speeding bullet. I often ask myself, "Why did this have to happen to me, and why at this time in my life?"

After reaching over 10,000 followers on Instagram, life was headed in a fast, but upward direction. 2020 has been the best, but yet at the same time, the worse year of my life. Keep reading and you will find out how life has a crazy sense of humor and a way of changing your daily routine as if it never existed.

Some things in life we just can't see coming, and won't ever be prepared for. The only thing guaranteed in life is that we will all die one day. The question is; what will you have accomplished before that day comes? As a human being, what did you contribute to this planet? That's what leaving a legacy is all about. At some point in life, we all learn from a lesson our ancestors left behind. What lesson will our generation of people teach the next?

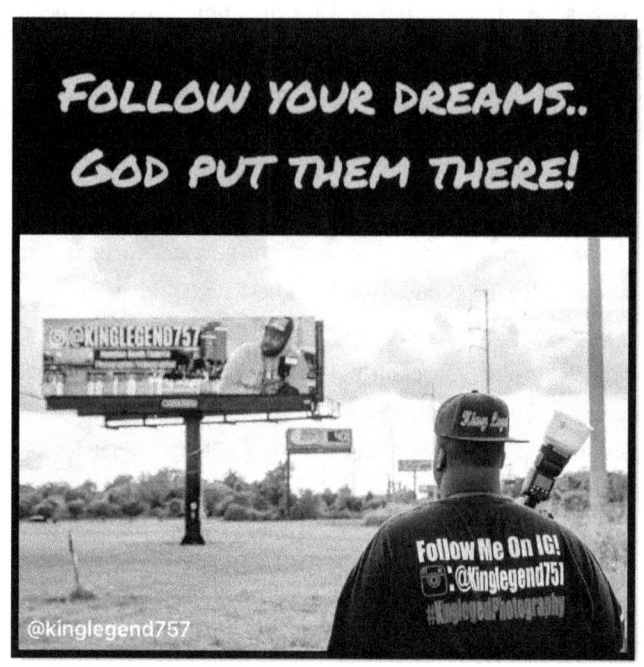

Chapter Two – LIFE OR DEATH

I remember it like it was a piece from a movie. It started after a weekend of fun, spending time with family at my house. Not a big crowd, no more than eight of us in total. On the first day, I had a temperature of 102 degrees. I was very hot and started to feel light-headed. All I wanted to do was lay down and rest my body.

I really didn't think much of it, I assumed that maybe I just had a fever and that it would go away within a day, at the most two. It was two days later when I decided to go to Med Express to get checked out. Of course, the coronavirus was new at this time back at the beginning of March. The rumor was still that only the elderly people with underlined health conditions were in danger of catching the virus.

After I checked in with the Doctor at the facility, they gave me an x-ray of my chest. The results came back that I had bronchitis. They gave me a prescription to go pick up medicine from the store. It was getting late and all the pharmacies were closing early due to the pandemic. By the time I left to go get my medication, the pharmacy was already closed.

However, I felt as if they diagnosed me wrong because I wasn't showing any of the signs of bronchitis. I had zero coughs and was only showing symptoms of a fever. I remember asking them for a Covid-19 test, and at that time they were only available to extremely sick patients, who showed signs of shortness of breath, fever, and people who had come in contact with others who had the virus already.

So of course, I was denied the test. Two days later went by after I had left Med Express, diagnosed with bronchitis. My fever had increased in temperature to 103 degrees and for the first time, I started to feel extremely weak. I was taking Tylenol trying to lower the fever for the entire week and nothing would break it.

I had my wife treating me with a damp washrag, patting my forehead with it, just trying to cool me down. My entire body felt like a furnace, but yet I did not break a sweat. Then that's when I started to feel as if all the oxygen in the room had just left. I was stuck laying in the bed for a total of 4 days with a fever.

I remember telling my wife to go to sleep in our guest room because I didn't want her to catch whatever it was I had. So we distanced ourselves living in the same house. She occasionally came into the room to check on me, as a good nurse would. Then she would leave to go back into the other room.

I just knew whatever it was I was feeling was completely different from anything my body had ever encountered before. I decided to go to Riverside hospital to get a second opinion on my situation. Of course, I had my wife drive me there, and she had to wait in the car.

Every step I took towards the hospital door felt like I could collapse at any moment. After the prescreening in the main lobby, they placed me in a room and began to give my body fluids. The Doctor told me that Extra Strength Tylenol should help with my fever and along with getting my body hydrated with fluids, I should be good to go. They had successfully got my temperature down to 98 degrees for the first time in a week almost.

After the temperature went down, I was discharged from the hospital and sent back home. That same day almost by the time I made it back home, my fever came back to pay me a visit. This time the temperature shot all the way up to almost 104 degrees. I remember becoming very frustrated and continued to take the Tylenol.

At this point my wife had ice packs on my body in rotation, placing them on my arms and chest area trying to cool me down. This was the most miserable feeling ever. Imagine just soaking in discomfort. The next day was one of the most challenging of the week. The news had announced that Sentara Hospital was giving free Covid-19 test to people.

I remember driving up and waiting in this long line, just to be denied a test. One of the nurses issuing the test told me that because I was young that even if I had the virus, it would just go away, and that they had to preserve the test for people who truly needed them because they had a limited amount of available test. I had already been seen by the hospital two times in one week.

On both visits, I was sent home without a clear answer on what was going on. Whatever it was, I knew it clearly had to be more than a fever and bronchitis. The next day is when my body would stop holding down food. I remember trying to force myself to eat a pizza from Papa John's. I took maybe two or three bites and instantly vomited.

Later that day, I tried eating chicken noodle soup and the same result. At this point my fever was still present, I was experiencing extreme nausea, shortness of breath, vomiting, and this feeling as if I could pass out at any moment. I remember stepping outside in my backyard for about 20 minutes, just to see if getting fresh air a little bit would help. That day was very breezy outside as if it was about to storm. The wind felt great against my heated body and I started to feel a little better.

As soon as I went back into the house it was as if sickness was alive in the bedroom. I could feel it come right back on me as if I was putting on a jacket. The time was around 4pm and I remember my wife looking so worried about what I was going through.

I kept telling her, I was going to be fine, but she insisted I go back to the Hospital. I remember telling her many times throughout that day that I was not going to go back to the hospital because I felt that they were not going to do anything for me.

I had already been twice and basically, all they would have me do is wait to be seen, and then discharge me within 20 minutes. I grew tired of going through the waiting process and having to struggle to get from point A to point B. After many conversations of me being stubborn and telling her no, this feeling came over me while I was lying down as if I had to vomit.

I started to dry heave and felt my saliva sitting on the bottom of my tongue. I immediately rushed to the master bathroom upstairs next door to my room and somehow feeling as if I was sleepy or tired. I wanted to be close to the toilet in case I needed to vomit, so I ended up lying down on the bathroom floor.

That was how my wife found me when she came back upstairs. She immediately said to me, "Either you're going to the hospital right now, or I am calling the ambulance." I had no more fight left in me and I knew she was serious, so I agreed to go to the hospital a third time. This time I decided to go to Sentara CarePlex in Hampton, VA to be evaluated.

They were prescreening patients outside the hospital in a little tent-like structure. I remember being so weak that they actually had to roll me inside with the help of a wheelchair from the car. This was bad, much worse than all the other trips taken to the hospital.

My memory starts to get a little blurry because everything happened so fast after being seen by a Doctor. He informed me that, I had double pneumonia in my lungs and a respiratory infection. He also told me that I showed all the signs of someone who has the coronavirus and that there was no cure for it at this time. He soon recommended that I be put on a ventilator to give my body a rest and that my chances of making it were not very high if I were to go back home.

I was barely making out the words that were coming out of his mouth; due to the fact, my body was extremely weak. I remember my wife being beside me, crying as she heard what the doctor had to say because she felt as if they were going to send me back home again.

I had a hard time processing how I went from feeling completely fine a week before this, and now dealing with life-threatening symptoms. I didn't grow up going to the hospital much. I had literally just been to the hospital more in this one week than I had been in my entire life.

The irony of the situation was I did not know what a ventilator was, and when the doctor told me that was basically my only option; I just replied, "O.K." I then signed a document stating that I was going to accept the treatment.

I remember a moment of silence as I was in the hospital room by myself, and all of a sudden I felt the need to contact my loved ones and let them know what was going on.

I don't know why, but the first person I called was my uncle who is a pastor. He began to pray over my health and then I called my wife and told her to call him. I wanted her to keep in contact with him while I was out because I wanted her to be strong mentally for me. Before I knew it another Doctor came into the room with this long tube-like thing. I felt like I was becoming Darth Vader from a Star Wars movie or something.

I had no clue what a ventilator was, but I was about to get a crash course real quick. The only thing I can truly remember was the pain of the tube getting shoved in through my nose and the Doctor telling me to swallow. With every swallow, the Doctor shoved the tube deeper up my nose, until it went all the way down to the back of my throat. I still can't believe I was actually awake during this process.

It was the most uncomfortable feeling I have ever had in my life. Just imagine feeling as if you are choking, but have to get comfortable with that pain. No matter how long I had that tube down my throat, my body was never able to get comfortable.

There was no getting used to that feeling at all. I just remember having to trust that the Doctors knew what they were doing and that I was not the first patient that had to go through this. That's what I normally tell myself to build confidence when dealing with situations of the unknown. I really don't remember much about this next part, other than it was time for the final step in the process.

A doctor came into the room and said to me, "Alright Mr. Campbell, we are going to be putting you to sleep now." I remember for the first time, actually being nervous. Not being sure if it would be the last time I would see anybody or even wake up after this procedure.

I also remember being very confident that everything was going to be fine and I would get through this. I have always been a firm believer in Jesus Christ, and have always lived my life with the attitude that he got me back regardless of the circumstances of any situation. My faith in God was all the confidence I needed to have hope.

In the next part of this book, I will take you through this crazy dream that was very dark and ugly, more like a nightmare. This is the part of my story that gets a little crazy and still gives me the creeps to this day. Some of it, I don't know if I was dreaming or if it was really happening. I will explain my entire dream for the first time in the next chapter.

People often ask me when I was asleep did I dream about anything. I always tell them yes, but never go into detail about what it was I dreamed about because it gives me the chills because I don't understand the meaning. It was basically a nightmare that seemed to go on forever, so much death of people I knew, but a weird feeling of peace that I still can't explain. It literally could be a Hollywood Film.

THIS WAS THE LAST PHOTO I SENT MY WIFE BEFORE I WAS PUT TO SLEEP.

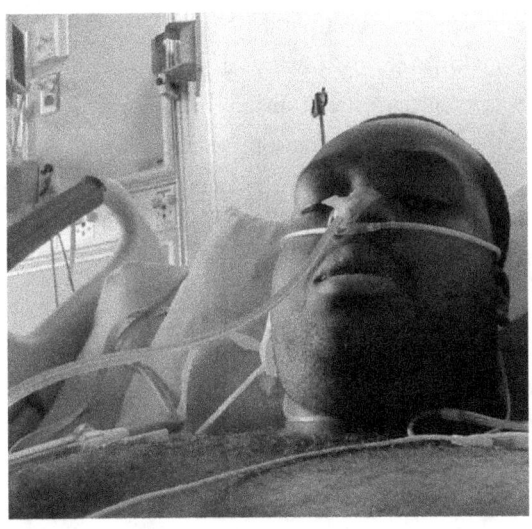

"Imagine feeling as if you are choking, but can't do anything about it. You have to become comfortable with feeling uncomfortable."

Chapter Three – Dream or Reality

While writing this book and discussing some of the gore details of my dreams with my wife and close friends, I decided to leave out some of the extreme parts of my dream; due to the fact they involve real people that I know. Out of respect to them, I will keep their role in my dream anonymous. Also after deep thought, I realized that I had multiple dreams and not just one long extended dream. I just couldn't process the information at that time because; I literally slept through all of it.

However, my dreams felt so real, I couldn't tell you if I was awake or asleep. In my first dream, someone who was trying to hold me ransom kidnapped me, in hope that my brother who owed him money would pay up in exchange for my life. I have no clue as to why I would have such a crazy dream.

When I tell you the dream felt so real, I could look around the apartment and even smell scents. I remember the anger on the kidnapper's face and how he wanted to do me harm. In the dream, the kidnapper drugged me to make me extremely weak and less aware of my surroundings so I wouldn't be able to put up a fight.

Eventually, in my dream, my brother-in-law kicked in the door and rescued me from the kidnapper. That is a watered-down version of my first dream, for the sake of your time and sanity. In my second dream, I truly can't explain too many details because of the amount of death in my dream of people I know.

The only information I can tell you is, it was a continuation of my first dream. If it were a movie I would title it, "The Kidnapper Strikes Back." In this dream, apparently, a lot of people were upset that I managed to escape with the help of my brother-in-law, and it was handled in a Mexican Cartel style ambush on my family.

In this dream, I lost two close people to me and I somehow managed to survive after being shot in my right arm and having my legs brutally damaged by someone trying to join a gang. In this dream, I was rescued and sent away to a safe house. In my third dream, I was at the safe house and all the security that was there to protect me ended up losing their lives to people coming to kill me.

I ended up coming face to face with the person my brother owed money to, and somehow the guy had me confused and thought I was my brother. I remember trying to explain to him that I was the wrong person and that I didn't know who he was and definitely didn't owe him money.

For some reason, he wanted to torture me and kill me slowly. Just before I was about to be executed, my brother arrived, and I remember him telling the guy, "That's my little brother, let him go. I am the one you want." The guy responded to him, "That was good of you to show up, that took to heart.

Too bad, not enough heart to stop me from shooting you right now." Then he shot my brother right there in front of me and offered me a chance to join him, or have the same fate as my brother. Even though now I know it was a dream, at that time I felt all the emotions as I was experiencing it.

I truly believed all of the deaths were real and that this nightmare was a reality. Again, I really don't understand why I had such crazy dreams, and honestly hope to never understand them. Also, keep in mind; this is a watered-down version of the details of my dream for your time and sanity.

I am summarizing the events in my dreams to the best of my ability, without losing the key factors that will explain my actions later on after I woke up. This next dream was the strangest of them all. It was like a scene cut out of a Mr. Scrooge, A Christmas Carol movie.

In my fourth dream, I attended my own funeral. I saw my parents sitting in the front row. My mother was crying and leaning on my father's shoulder. I remember seeing my dad who has always been this fearless, firm, and emotionless person shed one tear from his eye. He was very strong and stood on the belief that I was in a better place. I remember seeing my brothers, aunts, and uncles all in attendance.

They looked so real as if they were right in front of me and I could see the emotion on their faces. The dream started off with me lying down in the coffin. Then all of a sudden like a ghost, I came out of my body and saw myself lying down inside the coffin.

After seeing who was at the funeral and observing their emotions, I began to go up. I traveled all the way up through the clouds at a speed I can't even explain. When I came to a stop, I remember seeing this bright light and my grandmother who had just passed away on November 8, 2019. She didn't say anything to me, I just remembered looking at her face and saw a big smile.

Then she waved at my as if she was saying goodbye, I'll see you later. Then the weirdest thing happened in my dream; I woke up in the hospital and remember seeing a show on the TV in my room. It was a video of some preacher who was talking about how Jesus died for our sins and explaining how he saved us on the cross.

At this point, I could not tell you if I was dreaming or if I was really up in the hospital watching this show with my own eyes, but I remember praying to God that if he helped me get out of this situation, I promised to always put him first in everything I do. Then in my dream, I remember going back to sleep and waking up to this Doctor who was running a test on me.

I was very disoriented and not aware of this long plastic tube-like object that was hanging out of my nose. So I began to pull it and more of it started to come out until it turned red with blood coming out of my nose. The Doctor immediately told me not to pull on that and that it needed it to be where it was at.

After that happened I fell back asleep and woke back up in my hospital bed. The rest of my dreams actually took place from the hospital setting. I remember waking up and a nurse telling me that my wife was in the next room and that she had a minor headache and fever. The doctor also told me congratulations on my wife being pregnant with a baby.

I do not remember if she said it was a girl or boy. Honestly, that medication that the hospital gives you when they put you to sleep is so strong! If you had told me this same stuff before me being drugged, I immediately would have known what was true and not true. It was like; whatever my mind thought was real, ended up being real to me in my own world!

So let's recap real quick, I had all these dreams about me being kidnapped, rescued, attending my own funeral, visiting my grandmother in heaven, finding out my wife is pregnant, family members being killed, and on top of all that, me surviving life-threatening events.

If that doesn't sound like an insane adventure then I don't know what does. Now that I look back, I notice that all my dreams were extremely emotional encounters. I also had a few more dreams, but for the sake of this book and people interested in only my encounter with the coronavirus, I will move on.

From this point on in my story, I will be off of the ventilator explaining to you the moments, I was hallucinating in the hospital. Soon you will understand why I titled this chapter, "Dream or Reality." When I first became aware that I was off of the ventilator, it felt as if I had just woke up from a deep sleep. In my mind, not even a day had passed since the last time I remembered falling asleep.

This memory starts off with me getting checked on by a doctor asking me questions. "Do you know what year it is? Who is the President of the United States? What is your birthday? How many fingers am I holding up?" After asking me those questions, the Doctor began to explain to me that I had Covid-19 and that I was very sick.

I remember trying to explain to the Doctor that I was in the hospital was because I had been shot. It's so crazy to me how the stuff that happened to me in my dream, could fit every explanation that I had. I remember my right arm being weak and not being able to lift it up, as a Doctor was trying to check my blood pressure.

She needed to put the sleeve around my arm and I explained to her that I could not lift it. She said, "What happened to your arm, Mr. Campbell? I responded, "I can't lift that arm because that's where I got shot, and now the nerves are bad." Obviously to me, I still thought my dream was real and it made perfect sense for my arm to not respond because in my dream I had an experience where I actually got shot in my arm.

The Nurse responded, "Oh my goodness, I'm so glad you are alive. You are truly a miracle." I realize now that she was really telling me that she was happy I made it off the ventilator. Unfortunately, my mind took her response as confirmation of what I had said was true, and that I really was NOT dreaming.

So I began to process, all the people who had died in my dreams including my brother. I remember trying to explain to every Nurse what I had just gone through and how I just survived the most bloody events life can throw at you.

I also remember telling them that my brother had got shot right in front of me, and how my wife was pregnant in the next room. I would tell every nurse to go tell my wife in the next room that, I love her.

They would always ask, "Your wife is in the next room?" Then they would say, OK and leave the room. Ha-ha, I'm sure by now they really knew I was hallucinating and was just literally losing my mind. Seems to be a normal thing for people that come off of that medication. One of the side effects should read: May cause you to talk crazy and believe stuff that does not exist.

One night in the hospital, I remember thinking one of the nurses was in trouble. I heard a loud scream coming from the nurse booth outside of my room and I tried to disconnect all of the stuff from my arm and hop out of the bed to go run to the rescue. That was a big mistake. As soon as my feet hit the ground, I collapsed right to the floor and couldn't pick myself back up.

An alarm went off in my room and immediately nurses came rushing in telling me that I was not allowed to get out of the bed. I believe they ended up strapping me down to the bed and placed this camera in my room to observe my movements if I tried to get up. An alarm would sound off if I moved too far off of the mattress.

For the first time in the hospital since waking up, I became aware that there was something wrong with my body. I was extremely weak and could not even sit up using my own strength. I could not stand and I also had slurred speech. I looked down at this bag connected to my penis and remember not being able to turn over on my side without the help of a nurse.

When I had to use the bathroom, I had this pan the nurse would slide under me, so I could handle my business right in bed. I remember them coming in to clean me up and wipe me clean as they do for the elderly. That feeling I would not wish on anybody. Especially with me being only 26 years old, the last thing I wanted was another person wiping my behind.

Some things in life are meant to be private. Nevertheless, I ended up adapting and knowing that the nurses were just doing their jobs for my own good. I truly thank God for people like them and their service. You have to really have a passion for what you do in a job like that.

On top of me giving them a very hard time with my hallucinations.

I have to tell you guys about this one crazy hallucination that is so weird. I remember waking up with a nurse telling me that I was being transported by helicopter to a facility in New York to run tests on me. I was informed that they needed to draw blood and then I would fly right back.

The crazy part about this hallucination was I felt the room shaking as if I really was on a helicopter. I remember arriving at the Sentara Hospital in New York City, and when we arrived my nurse turned my television to the show titled, "THE GAME."

I had never watched this show before and remember being hooked on the episode I saw that day. I remember watching two entire episodes before a nurse came into my room to draw blood. After she finished, the helicopter started to shake and I was on my way back to Sentara Hospital in Hampton, VA.

Later on, I will explain why this was so crazy and still sometimes give me the chills. My moment of truth in the hospital did not come to me until I was able to speak to my wife on the phone for the first time. In our first conversation, I literally was trying to tell her about everyone who had, died, and how I was sorry for not being there with the baby, and how I am sorry for missing our anniversary.

She kept trying to tell how everything was fine and that nobody died. I didn't snap out of it until I told her I saw my brother get shot right in front of me, and I was there when he died. She responded, "Deion, you were put to sleep for twelve days. None of that stuff happened.

Your brother is doing fine, I just talked to him earlier; he just wants you to get better." Then it hit me; all of that stuff I thought I was experiencing was a dream! I felt such a relief come over me, that I started crying. To me, three people just came back alive from the grave, and it was the happiest moment in my life.

At one point in the hospital, I could not hold down any food. Whatever they gave me, I would vomit it moments later. They put me on a liquid type diet in the beginning and eventually I progressed to eating graham crackers with apple juice.

I remember a nurse coming into the room to check on my speech and to see if I could swallow my crackers down. I did that for a few days and then they said I could eat regular food. I don't remember them ever taking the tube out of my nose. They must have done it when I was asleep. If that is the case, I am thankful for that.

I wouldn't want to imagine the pain of getting that tube out of my throat and out through my nose. So to recap, at this point I am aware that I was hallucinating in the hospital and my family was safe. For the first time, I can truly say my nerves were calmed down back to normal, and I could start to function and have my mind back as the medication wore off. Now at this part in the process, I could tell the nurses were happy about my success at beating the virus.

I was introduced to Doctor Olsen who was my primary Doctor helping me while I was asleep on the ventilator. This Doctor saved my life in my opinion. I know it was a team effort, but I can't overlook how much passion she has for her patients. I could tell that she really wanted everything to work out for me and had my best interest at heart.

She would come just to check up on me and always kept her word when she said she was going to do something. That trust and the bond we established, meant the world to me. She was that hope that radiated whenever she entered the room. Always bringing me good news about how I was doing so much better than before. It was her attitude that made my recovery so smooth, along with a combination of me wanting to go back home and see my family.

I wanted to get out of the hospital so bad. Not because of the nurses, but because I was literally lying down on the bed every minute of the day. All I could do is watch Television. I remember my favorite shows to watch that made my time go by were Pawn Stars, Bar Rescue, The Parkers, Martin, American Pickers, and Blackish. Those shows literally got me through the long hours of the day.

Due to the coronavirus, the entire world was shut down, and there were no visitors allowed in the hospital. That made things 10x as hard to deal with because for almost an entire month, I was not able to see one familiar face that I knew. All the staff was instructed to wear hospital protective gear and mask when entering a room. So technically, I didn't even know what any of my nurse's face looked like. I thank God that they were good at their job.

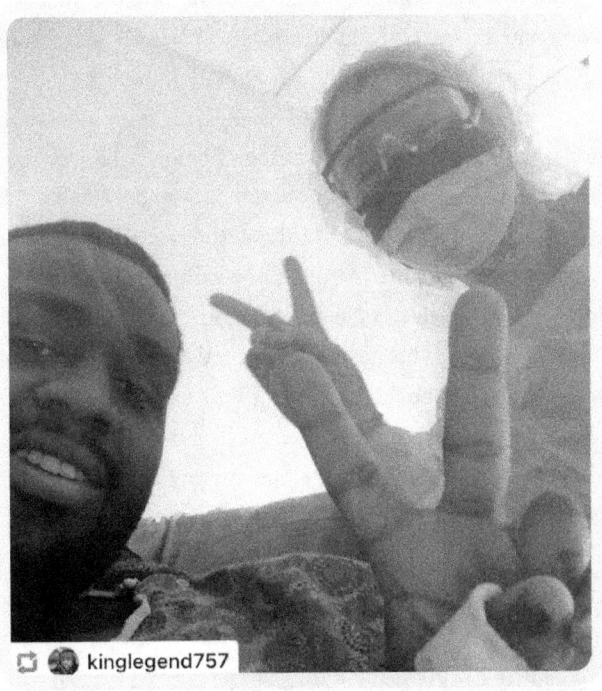

This is a selfie-photo taken of Doctor Olsen and I after a long fight to get me back to a stable condition and feeling good.

Chapter Four – DEJA VU

While I was on the ventilator, my body went through a tremendous amount of stress. The fever I had did not break for days. It eventually caused my other body organs to have complications. Such as kidney functions, liver, and blood clots in my lungs. We also can't forget double pneumonia my body was already fighting.

I know people who have died from pneumonia alone, with no other complications. I believe the Doctors at the hospital treated every problem as they developed. That is truly the only way to fight the coronavirus because there is no cure at this time. At one point on the ventilator, I had an aspiration from the feeding tube, in which fluid went up from my stomach because it wasn't traveling where the tube was supposed to be feeding me.

I received a miracle; there is no doubt about that. My fever finally broke, and somehow my body managed to endure the fight against all of those symptoms at the same time. After coming off of the ventilator, which I was on for twelve days, my body had to gain its motor functions back again. Your muscles in your body are working out daily even when you don't think they are.

If you were to all of a sudden not use them, you would start to lose strength in them. This is why astronauts workout when they travel out in space. The lack of gravity makes them light as a feather. So if you are lying down for too long your body is fighting less gravity, and in return so is your muscles. After having my body lay down for almost two weeks, I had very little strength and was so weak, even rolling over in my bed was a challenge.

I remember one of the first things being treated when I came off of the ventilator was my feet. Apparently, after laying down so long, I had developed pressure ulcers on my feet, which were very ugly, and not attractive at all to watch. They looked like a football that had been chewed up by a vicious animal.

I had fluid build up on the ankle of my left foot, almost the size of a tennis ball. I was instructed to let it drain on its own and not to burst it. The pain on the bottom of my feet made it almost impossible to walk. As the medication wore off, the pain level started to rise. I started to feel a lot more than before. I had a throbbing pain in my shoulder around my collarbone area, which made it impossible to get comfortable.

This pain was very sharp and seemed to never stop. I remember being so happy when they told me, I would be seen by a physical therapist. That information to me meant I would be getting out of the hospital soon. Little did I know, how much therapy I actually needed. My first therapy session was very simple, but it helped me realize the reality of how weak I actually was.

The therapist entered the room and told me that today all he wanted me to focus on was sitting up. He adjusted the bed and then assisted me in the sitting position.

Immediately the entire room began to spin and I had a throbbing headache. I used so much energy just to get to that position. I sat up for about 90 seconds and then I returned to my original position in the bed.

We attempted this about two times and that was the end of my first therapy session. I remember being short-winded after that first session, breathing as if I had just run down the hallway. That was a feeling, I would soon learn would become a new normal in my daily life. In the second therapy session, we attempted the same routine and added a few stretches. We also began rotating the arms and bending the legs. Eventually, therapy progressed to me attempting to stand up with the help of two therapists.

I remember my first time standing; I was in disbelief how hard it was to do. It was so painful, I felt as if my feet were fighting me instead of supporting me as usual. I was determined to fight back and not let the pain win. My attitude came from a place in my mind where I was telling myself, I'm too young for this. I have to move on, this can't be how the rest of my life will be.

I only managed to stand for about 30 seconds with their help, but we tried it many more times in the therapy sessions to come. Eventually, I gained back the strength to do it on my own. The next phase of my therapy was one of the most challenging. I had to learn to take baby steps with the use of a walker.

On the first day, I remember taking about three steps before I felt exhausted and out of breath. We did not give up and my therapist always praised whatever amount of progress I was making. That definitely helped build my confidence, and eventually, all I wanted to do was make my physical therapist proud. I felt as if he was bragging about me to the other staff.

Eventually, therapy transitioned to me being able to put on my own socks and being able to sit out of the bed on the couch next to it. I had a very hard time adjusting to sitting down versus lying down in the bed. Sitting down had become a challenging task and hard to do with the pain I was constantly feeling in my shoulder. The pain increased almost double when I was sitting. I remember they would tell me to sit for 15-30 minutes. I hated it so much; I was in so much pain.

I was also still attached to the alarms, so I couldn't move without causing a scene in the hospital. So I had to just tough it out and make the best out of it. The thoughts, that were going on in my mind at that time were just trying to process how my body got to that condition.

I was just fine traveling the country, taking photos of concerts, walking, talking, and getting around with no problems on my own two feet. I felt as if I could deal with it differently if I knew what I had done to cause this pain. Like, if I had been in a car accident I could say the reason I am struggling to walk is that a car hit me.

It was hard for me to process not being able to walk normally because I had a new virus called the coronavirus. I believe the hardest part of having Covid-19 was the lack of experience people had with dealing with patients in my condition. It was almost impossible to get a clear answer when you had a question about your health.

So I had to be very understanding, the Doctors and I were learning about my coronavirus together. This global pandemic had taken the world by storm. Luckily for the United States, we were one of the last countries to experience it. We as a nation had other countries to learn from based on how they handled it.

However, even with looking at other countries' experiences with Covid-19, there were still too many unanswered questions out there to provide any solid answers to patients dealing with the virus. So I was basically in a situation where I could not see the road ahead because many had not traveled the road to recovery in my condition yet.

I guess that is why everyone considered me to be a miracle. Healthwise there were a lot of things that could have easily made me another coronavirus statistic adding to the already rising number of deaths in the country. People who have not experienced the virus or who may not know anyone personally with the virus have no clue how serious the virus really is.

I hear people so quick to scream it's not really a virus going on, or it's just a government conspiracy trying to scare people. To me regardless of what you think it may be, this virus we are all dealing with is REAL. If we do not mature as citizens in this country and put the health of the people living in it first, we will never stop the spread of a virus that has proven to kill people all over the world.

People have to understand until we find a cure for this virus, the only thing we can do is try to stop the spread of it. That is the reason they are encouraging social distancing. It's not because staying at home will stop you from getting the virus, it's because it will significantly decrease your chances of catching it; or if you already have it and don't know it, spreading it to someone else.

A lot of people ask me in interviews if I think the world should open back up and proceed back to normal. I honestly don't have an answer to that question. There are no making people happy, in a world that runs by the use of currency. You know what they say, "Money makes the world go around." Which is more important to the government, is it the economy or the people who live in it? I know which one is more important to me.

All I want in this world is for people to be happy and be able to live out their dreams. Nobody should have to worry about catching a virus, every time they go out in public to spend time with their family. Unfortunately, this is now the world we live in. For now, all we can do is respect our neighbor's boundaries and try to keep each other safe.

At first, people thought only the elderly people with underlined health issues could catch the virus. I am a living coronavirus survivor testament to that is not true. People are catching this virus at all ages. All we can do is try to do is prevent the ones we love from catching it, by washing our hands more frequently and keeping our environment clean. I wouldn't wish Covid-19 on my worse enemy.

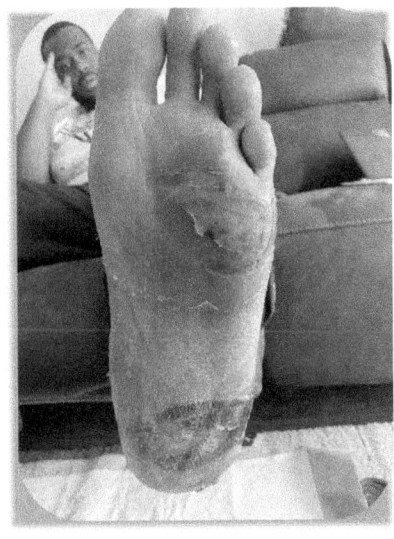

This is what my feet looked like as they were healing up. Believe it or not, they actually looked worse than this, before treating them.

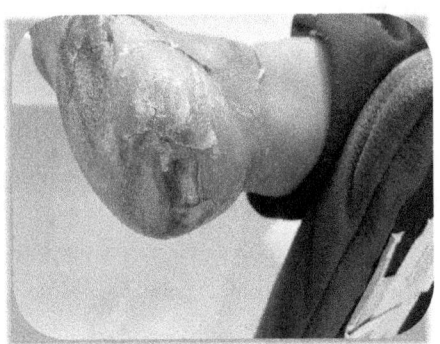

No I am not a diabetic, nor did I have issues with my feet before Covid-19.

Chapter Five – Road To Recovery

The road to recovery is a challenge mentally, physically, and spiritually. There are many bumps and potholes in it. While you are traveling it to reach your destination in life, it is also still under construction. I was amazed at how important the little things in life are to us. It's so easy to take for granted how special it is just to have two arms, two legs, two feet, and a brain that functions well. One change in any of those factors in your life and immediately, the lifestyle you are used to living has a whole new perspective. I had no clue that having Covid-19 could have such a vigorous effect on me.

Coming off of the ventilator was just the beginning of the road ahead. A lot of people forget that going to the hospital is just part of the process. The recovery phase is just as important. My wife received so much support when I was on the ventilator fighting for my life. Phone calls every day, people sending gifts over to the house, random ghost shoppers dropping groceries at the door, enormous amounts of prayer, and more.

The moment the news got out that I survived and was off the ventilator, people sent their praises and that was the last we heard from many. I thank God for the people who still show their support, now that it is confirmed I am among the living and not the dead.

One of the most humbling experiences for me in the hospital was having another person clean me up with baby wipes after I used the bathroom. It felt as if I was a baby all over again, but with the knowledge of a grown man. Men don't want the feeling of someone wiping their behind. If that won't humble you, I don't know what will.

I remember vomiting like clockwork after I ate meals in the hospital when I first attempted to eat regular food. Nurses had to come and clean me up often. I know some of them had to get tired of visiting my room to clean me up, but they did their job and did not complain.

The only thing I could do was keep apologizing because I was not able to promise that I would not do it again. If any nurses that treated me are reading this book, I would like to thank you very much for putting up with me in the hospital. Over March and April, I spent more time with the staff of Sentara Hospital more than my own family.

We joked, laughed, and enjoyed each other company. You all inspired me to believe I am a miracle and gave me the positive energy I desperately needed around me to promote a successful recovery. Lord knows, it was very hard to watch TV in the Hospital.

Every commercial was about the coronavirus. I definitely couldn't watch the news because all they talked about was about how the numbers were going up daily and spiking an all-time high in certain cities.

I heard the word Covid-19 at least 100 times a day on television. The mental struggle was real to get my mind off of death. I couldn't help but ask myself, "Why am I still alive?"

All I saw on the television were people dying from catching the virus. It is truly a blessing for me to be alive. At the same time as seeing the crisis display on television, I was also not able to see my family. No visitation really played a hard part on me. The feeling of being lonely and forgotten about was constant.

You truly feel the 24 hours in your day, when the only thing you can do is lay down in one room. I couldn't even change the scenery. I hadn't felt the wind blow up against my skin or even the heat from the sun for at least a month.

The food at the hospital was very healthy, to say the least. Absolutely, no flavor in any of the meals delivered to my room. It was like salt was banned from the hospital and also from my diet. It was the same fate for anything sweet as well, zero sugar in all drinks. This was quite an adjustment for a guy like me who was over 400 pounds.

I dropped almost 50 pounds in the two weeks I was on the ventilator. That was a very fast weight loss, which is expected to happen to someone as sick as I was. One of the things I fell in love with at the Hospital was iced cold water. I remember feeling so dehydrated when I first got off of the ventilator.

It felt as if I had not had a drop of water in my system for over ten years. Even though the doctors were giving me plenty of fluid through the IV, I just couldn't get rid of the feeling of being thirsty. I used to ask the nurse for water so much in the hospital that they used to refer to me as the water boy.

Some of the nurses working used to just bring me, two pitchers of water, at a time. Eventually, they would bring me 2 pitchers of water and one pitcher of ice. Honestly, I would ask the nurses for so much water because I could not get up and get myself some water from the sink. I was in a way handcuffed to the bed.

I had to rely on the nurse on duty for everything. Another beverage that I became obsessed with in the hospital was apple juice and milk. Apple Juice was the only beverage that tasted like it had sugar in it and for some odd reason, cold milk just made me feel refreshed. I also remember liking the orange juice a lot too.

One morning I drunk two cartons of milk and then followed it with one apple juice, immediately I vomited it all right back up like a baby. After that, I remember telling myself to never do that again.

Another thing I remember about my stay at the hospital was how gaining my speech back was a process. For some weird reason after detaching that tube from the throat, my tongue felt it weighed two pounds and it started to affect my speech. I sounded so terrible, I sounded like I had been out drinking and was far from sober.

Truly embarrassing, I remember calling a friend while I was hallucinating and leaving a long voicemail on the phone. I still haven't heard the voicemail and not sure if

I even want to. The front part of my tongue felt numb, which was making it hard to feel when it connected to teeth, which help to pronounce certain words.

That is why I also had a speech therapist come visit me to make sure I was gaining that motor skill back. I am so grateful I gained the bass back in my voice and it is back to normal now. It took a few weeks to get it back to normal. Another thing that I had to get used to was getting blood drawn. If you're not a fan of needles then this would really be a problem for you. I was getting blood drawn from me at least four times a day.

The Doctors ran many tests on me that required a sample of my blood for each one. The worse part about being in the hospital for me was waking up to the nurse turning my room light on at five o'clock in the morning telling me she needed to draw some blood.

I had been poked so many times in the same vein that sometimes, it stopped cooperating and they would have to find another one to draw blood from. By the time I was done with the hospital, I had plenty of bruises on my arm. Another phase in my recovery was the Doctor disconnecting the catheter from my penis.

I had been urinating through that tube whenever I had to go to the bathroom for about three weeks. Even in my sleep, I would use the bathroom without knowing it. I did not have to think about that process very much.

I remember when they first disconnected it, that night I was very paranoid about peeing in the bed. I'd be lying if I said I didn't do that at least once or even three times, maybe even more times than that. My body had gotten used to being on a carefree schedule and urinating in my sleep with no mess to clean up afterward.

I'm sure my wife is glad she has not had to experience that part of my recovery. I grew out of that phase by the use of a urinal container. It was basically a bottle that's kept within arms reach to urinate in.

While on the topic of my bladder, I remember the Doctors put me on these laxatives that were very strong and gave me the runs. I'm talking about the type of poop that had a timer on it. Either you were going to get your butt to a toilet or the seat you are sitting on will become it.

Part of being a patient in the hospital is actually being patient. Some things just can't wait though, when your body says it's time to go, then it's time to go. Hitting the, "I need a nurse button" on the side of your bed did not always save the day.

Nurses are very busy working on many patients and may not always be able to answer your call when you need them. They try their very best and may get to your room within twenty minutes of your call if you're lucky. Needless to say, I definitely pooped on myself a few times in the hospital when I was waiting for a nurse to come to my rescue.

My stomach was no match for the laxatives my doctor was giving me, so I started to refuse the medication. I found it very unpleasant to be lying down in my own feces waiting on a nurse to clean me up. Is this too much information? Well, this is the full behind the scenes of my Covid-19 story. I really went through all of this as part of my recovery process.

After getting my body functions back to normal such as, eating, drinking, bladder control, and being able to make progress with the hospital therapy, it was time to be sent off to a rehab facility. I remember the day of getting discharged from Sentara hospital. It was a bittersweet feeling.

I had truly become attached to a lot of the nurses who cared for me in that month. Wonderful personalities and faces I knew I would not remember because of them all wearing masks. They truly got me through in the times of me not being able to get visits from my family.

That chapter in my process was officially coming to a close, and a new chapter was now beginning. I remember them hooking me up to the stretcher to place me in the transport van. The breeze from that day touched my skin like a hug from Mother Nature.

The sun was shining in all its glory and I appreciated every bit of it. I looked out the window of the transport van as we were leaving and I saw a glimpse of Sentara Hospital getting smaller in my view. I was actually leaving the hospital, but somehow I felt as if I was leaving home.

The day of my arrival at my real home was very close. Soon all of this would be a memory in the story of my life that I am blessed to have another chance at. I was being transported to Sentara Rehabilitation Center, which was the same facility I used to visit my grandmother at before she passed a few months before me being in the hospital.

I never imagined myself being checked into the same facility as her months later. I remember walking in the same building just to check up on her, now it was as if she would be watching me down from heaven to check up on me. Haha, at least she already knew the staff I would be dealing with.

I was placed in a quarantine hall in the facility and kept away from the general population. When I finally made it to my room, I remember being happy to have a window that I could actually have a nurse open. I also had my own bathroom with a sit-down shower in it. The room was much bigger than my space at Sentara Hospital, and the bed felt much better too.

The best part of my first day at rehab was the dinner. THE FOOD HAD SALT IN IT!!! My taste buds went crazy and the sweet tea almost drove me insane!! After eating what felt like struggle meals for almost a month, I was truly happy. Whoever was in that kitchen was definitely doing what they were supposed to be doing with their life. They have no idea how much the food touched my soul and gave me my appetite back. I couldn't wait for my next meal. I felt like I was in a presidential suite at a five-star hotel. They even gave snacks, real junk food. I probably gained my first 5 pounds back in rehab.

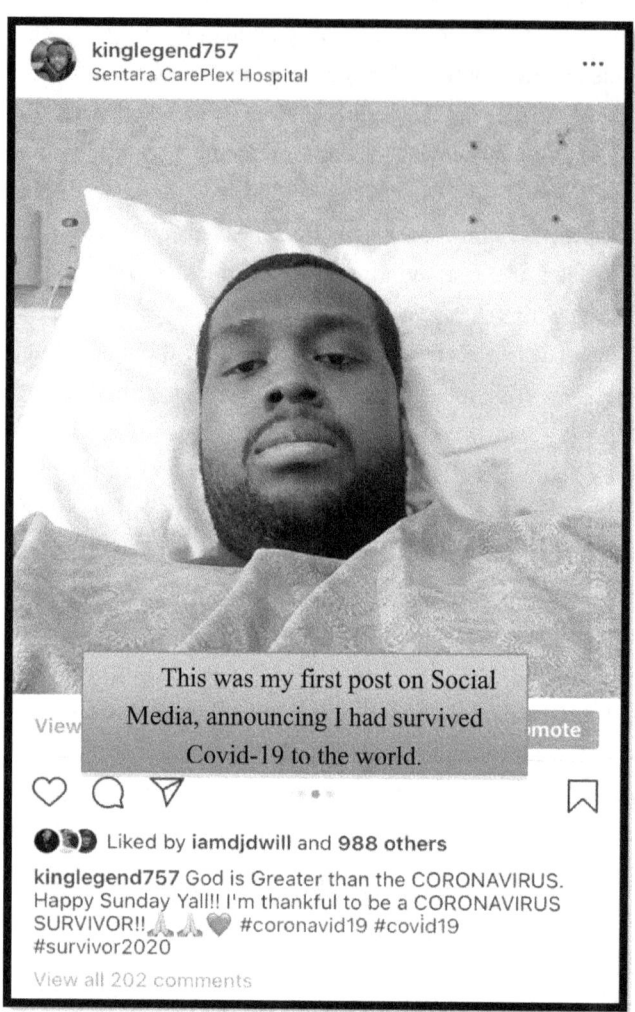

Chapter Six - Rehab

My first day in rehab was the first time since being in the hospital I was allowed to attempt to take a complete shower. All of the therapy I had previously leading up to this point, was all about gaining my motor skills back to a condition that could be trained. Rehab for me was all about being able to take care of myself without the assistance of another.

My first time in the shower, I remember sitting down trying my best to clean myself up. I was still weak and it took almost all the wind I had in me to do, but I gave it my best shot. My therapist assigned to me that morning had to finish washing me up in the shower.

One of the main problems I had to deal with in rehab was the constant pain in my feet from the pressure ulcers. I had so much fluid in my left ankle; I had to try my best not to put pressure on it. In the rehab, I was given a walker to help me get from my bedside to the bathroom. I remember my first time going to the bathroom on my own.

I was so happy that I could do it by myself, but something scared the heck out of me when I began to urinate. Blood was coming out of my penis instead of urine. It did not hurt, but it had a little sting feeling to it. I remember my heart dropping like what is wrong with me now! I didn't have this problem the entire time I was in the hospital. I then realized that this was the first time I was able to pee standing up without the use of a catheter.

I informed the nurse at the facility of what was going on with me and they reached out to my doctors at Sentara. They were informed that blood in my urine was normal because they had recently disconnected the catheter that was connected to my penis, but it should go away within the next day or two.

I was so relieved the first time I witnessed regular urine coming out of me instead of blood, it only took about 15-24 hours and I was back to normal. The staff at the rehab facility and I clicked immediately; as I was the youngest patient they had in the entire facility.

This rehabilitation center's primary patients were the elderly, almost like a nursing home set up. My favorite thing about the rehab facility other than the food was the staff. They truly bonded with me and treated me like family.

I got to meet every nurse on different shifts and all of them had a great sense of humor to go along with their jolly personalities. I remember joking with them about who was my favorite nurse.

On my first day in rehab, Janet Roach of channel 13 news who saw my post on Instagram about beating the virus contacted me. Andy Fox of Wavy News 10 also contacted me via Facebook trying to set up an interview about my experience.

Janet Roach was already following me on social media, so I decided to do the interview with her instead. We did the interview virtually through Instagram video chat right from my bed in the rehab. I felt really special after the interview because it made me feel connected for the first time to the outside world.

I remember turning the television set in my room to the news and watching my interview with Janet Roach on TV during primetime as an exclusive interview with Channel 13 news. The nurses at the rehab started to treat me like a celebrity at that point, even though they were already nice, to begin with.

They aired my story on every rotation of the news for a least a day. It was about day two in the rehab when I was tested again for the Covid-19 virus. To my surprise, the results came back positive! This was very disturbing news to me because I couldn't figure out how in the world I tested positive for Covid-19 and I had just tested negative for the virus at the hospital I just left.

The Doctor at the rehab informed me that they gave me a false negative and that I still had the virus in my system. I was not looking forward to this news at all, especially since I had just told the entire Hampton Roads area on the local news that I was Covid-19 free. This information mentally crushed my spirits because I thought I was in the clear, not still fighting the virus.

The facility wasn't taking in Covid-19 positive patients, but in my case, they ended up having me isolated (which I already was anyway) and the nurses were instructed to not enter my room without wearing protective equipment such as a mask/face shield and they had to throw away their paper gowns as they left my room.

The physical therapist also stopped coming until they received clarification on what to do about my situation. After further investigation of my case, it turned out that I tested positive for antibodies in my system, and it could take up to 6 weeks for the virus to completely shed from my system. As in, I had beaten the virus already and was not fighting it anymore; it just had to finish shedding. That news was a huge relief to the facility and I for sure.

The highlight of my time in rehab was being able to see my family for the first time in over a month! My family was not able to come into my room, but the rehab was allowing window visits. The public was allowed to come to your room window and you could see them. It's not as good as a contact visit, but compared to not seeing a familiar face at all, it was everything!

My wife visited me almost daily the entire time I was in rehab. I would have to talk to her on the cell phone as she stood outside on the other side of my window. Speaking of cell phones, I thank God for the ability to facetime or video chat with people in 2020!

That definitely got me through on the days she was not able to visit me in person. It was killing me that I lived so close to the rehab facility. I was so close to home, but yet so far away at the same time. I started to become homesick and just wanted to lay down in my own bed, for the first time in over a month.

There was still no set date for me to be discharged from rehab yet, so for the time being I was in the unknown as to when I would be returning home. One of the things I liked to do in rehab was watching shows on Netflix from my phone. I remember becoming addicted to the show "Black Lightning." I watched the entire season all from my phone right there in rehab.

Along with the physical therapy and full-course meals, I started to gain my strength back at a rapid pace and my physical therapist told me that I was making so much progress that she believed I would be able to go home in a few days. Eventually, I was even able to get around without the use of a walker.

It was very painful because of the condition of my feet, but doable because of the strength I gained back in my legs. My feet had to be wrapped daily, all the walking I was doing in therapy started to cause the fluid to drain slowly from the womb on my left foot.

There were times they had to bleach my entire room because of me leaking a trail of blood from the bed to the bathroom. Nevertheless, this still was major progress compared to how I was doing in the hospital. About a day or two later after taking a physical ability test, I received a call from the person in charge of discharging me from the rehab facility.

I was told that I would be able to go home on Thursday, but they recommended I quarantine for 14 days before going back home and that they would allow me to finish my quarantine at the facility if I wanted to. I was so happy to tell my wife that information, but at the same time, we had a debate about me coming home still needing to quarantine.

I felt as if I had been in quarantine since I got off of the ventilator and did not want to stay in the hospital/rehab any longer. I was ready to go back to my own space. I really didn't want to stay another day in rehab, but instead of putting my family at risk of catching the virus, I decided to stay and finish my recommended quarantine at the rehab facility, which pushed my discharge date back almost another week.

Those extra days were the longest days ever. It was like time was playing a prank on me and stopped moving. Each minute of my day felt like an hour. I remember trying to sleep the days away, only waking up to shower, eat, and talk on the phone to my wife. After a long journey that started with a fever, double pneumonia, 12 days on a ventilator, kidney/liver functions acting up, salt/sugar-free food, lying down 24 hours a day in a bed, gaining back my speech, motor skills, and rehab, I was finally about to return home! I would be continuing my recovery process with outpatient therapy from my own house.

My last day in rehab was just as bittersweet as leaving Sentara Hospital. Once again, I had bonded with the staff and had gotten used to them, only to just say goodbye and probably never see them again. It was at 8 o'clock in the morning when I received the phone call from my wife letting me know she was outside to pick me up.

The nurses at the facility were so excited and happy for me, they kept coming to my room to visit me and wish me luck in my future. My physical therapist at the facility made sure she came in on her day off that morning just to say goodbye. As my bags were packed and I was about to leave the room, one of my nurses came into the room trying to get me to look outside of my window.

As I looked, I observed the entire staff of nurses from the facility holding up poster signs in a line cheering me on, wishing me luck, and reminding me how happy they were I made it out alive. When I went outside and got inside of my car, my wife slowly drove to the crowd of nurses and they handed me balloons and posters with all of them leaving a message for me to read later. It felt like an entire parade, just for me. Words can't explain how special that moment was for me. I recorded the entire moment and they aired the replay on the local news. I believe all of the nurses that I encountered from the time I was in the hospital until the time I was leaving rehab are truly angels. What nurses do in this country and all over the world is truly heroic! Not many people can say, they helped save somebody's life. That is a job reserved for heroes and guardian angels sent from heaven.

This was the post I made on social media after leaving the facility.

 kinglegend757
Sentara Nursing and Rehab Center

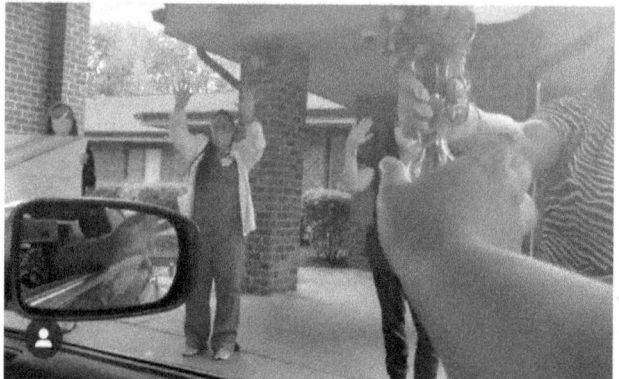

View Insights   Promote

1,039 views · Liked by **iamdjkarizma** and **tynitty757**
kinglegend757 Shoutout to all the Nursing Staff from Sentara Hospital and rehab center. They truly treated me like family and one of their own the entire 40+ days... more

View all 68 comments

Chapter Seven – Home Sweet Home

The feeling of getting in my car after a very long journey in the hospital and rehab was as if I had done two tours in Iraq and finally made it back to my family. The look on my wife's face was the emotion of true happiness. I had truly made it through the worse of my situation, with the help of God and so many caring people in my corner.

The entire time I was in the hospital, people were praying and even fasting for my recovery. As my wife pulled the car up in the driveway of my house, I remember the first thought that came to my mind was, I wonder if my dog Ricco would remember me. I told my wife to go inside the house first, and that I would walk in afterward to surprise Ricco.

When I stepped in through the door, I expected Ricco to act extremely excited to see me, but to my surprise, he was very scared as if he had just seen a ghost. I called his name and told him to come to me, but he just ran under my wife and tried to hide like a shy child does when being introduced to someone for the first time. Then it dawned on me that the reason he was acting this way was that he remembered the sound of my voice, but the look on my face had changed completely.

Before going to the hospital, I would keep my face clean-shaven, but for the first time ever, my dog was witnessing me with a full beard. I had not got a haircut in over a month. I attempted to pick him up to try and get him warmed up to my presence again, but he would just nervously lick my arm as I would pet him and hide the moment I placed him back on the ground.

The same day I came home, I had also called my barber to let him know that I needed an emergency haircut and that it would be a house call. He showed up later on that evening and gave me a fresh haircut right inside my garage. He was masked up, with gloves on, and ready for duty.

I remember being in so much pain trying to sit up straight because of the severe pain throbbing on my shoulder. There were a few times during the haircut that we had to take a break, just to give my shoulder a rest. I would have to lean forward with my elbows on my knees just to relieve the pain. However, my barber was very patient with me and was just happy I was alive and well.

He got the job done and I finally started to look healthy again. This was the first time I had ever had my beard grow out, so of course, my wife fell in love with the new look. My wife had decorated the house with a welcome home themed set up. There were balloons and a banner put up for me.

I remember when I was in the hospital; I told her that I wanted watermelon and my favorite steak, shrimp, and mash potatoes with gravy dinner when I came home. She kept her promise of course and that was exactly what I had for dinner that night. My mother-in-law joined us for dinner as we all celebrated my recovery. I believe that same week; I was contacted by Channel 13 news anchor Janet Roach, for a follow-up interview.

Once again, I was featured on the local news to talk about my experience with the coronavirus and to share a message of hope to those who may have contracted the virus-like me. I was truly blessed in my situation and still to this day give all the glory to God. I know without him watching over me, and the prayers from all the people exercising their faith, I would not be here.

The real prayer warriors truly showed up for me in my time of need, that's a fact. As I stated before, many people hear that a person made it out of the hospital, and without realizing it; they act as if the journey is now over. In reality, the hard work is just now beginning. When I first arrived home, I could walk on my own two feet, very slow. I was in a lot of pain and my feet had not completely healed yet.

I still had to have them wrapped daily by womb care who were coming to my house once a week to treat them and check my progress. I also had a physical therapist assigned to me so I could do outpatient therapy from home.

My house is two stories; so we had to focus on getting me able to climb the stairs to get to my bedroom, while at the same time protect the healing process of my feet. It was challenging at first, but as the days went on, my open wombs on my feet began to close and I was able to do more with my physical therapy.

The main challenge my physical therapist faced with dealing with me as a patient was trying to figure out a way to work the muscles in my right arm that we had no clue on exactly what was wrong with it. My right arm would not respond to any command to lift up. I could bend it like normal, but the lifting function was nonresponsive.

I remember trying to get an appointment set up for an MRI to be done, to hopefully get some answers, but facilities available dates were pushed back months at a time due to the government being shut down because of the coronavirus. Getting an appointment for almost anything at that time was a pain to do.

A lot of precautions were put in place to ensure the safety of the staff. At one point I was told I couldn't get an MRI because I had come in contact with Covid-19 and had to have two negative Covid-19 tests within 24 hours apart from each other. I began to become frustrated because I felt like I had an important need that wasn't being tended to because of my previous condition holding me back.

I didn't know much about nerve damage at that time, but my neurologist suspected after his evaluation, that would explain the issue going on with my arm. Not being able to lift my arm was life-changing to me because I needed it to also lift up my camera.

My daily life until the day of my MRI consisted of me waking up, going downstairs, sitting on the recliner sofa, playing the video game or watching Netflix, waiting on physical therapy, taking my medication, and after spending the entire day downstairs finally taking the trip back upstairs to get in the bed.

I repeated this process over and over again. Days turned into weeks and weeks turned into months. As much as I was happy to be alive, the quality of my life started to get to me. I started to lose myself; because this is not the person I remembered being. I started to feel useless and hated the feeling of needing help for everything.

I have always been ambitious and used every minute of my day to the fullest. At one point in my life, I didn't have time for video games or television. Now it seemed as if my life had flipped completely upside down and I had all the time in the world to do absolutely nothing at all.

This next chapter in my life was a very low point for me mentally. Keep reading and I am sure you will understand my pain. One thing about my experience with dealing with the virus, it taught me a lot about patience and how to be mentally strong. You know the saying, "What doesn't kill you, makes you stronger." Well, that applies to everything physically but also mentally! My mind was facing a challenge, as it had never encountered before.

THIS IS MY FIRST POST ON SOCIAL MEDIA AFTER RETURNING HOME.

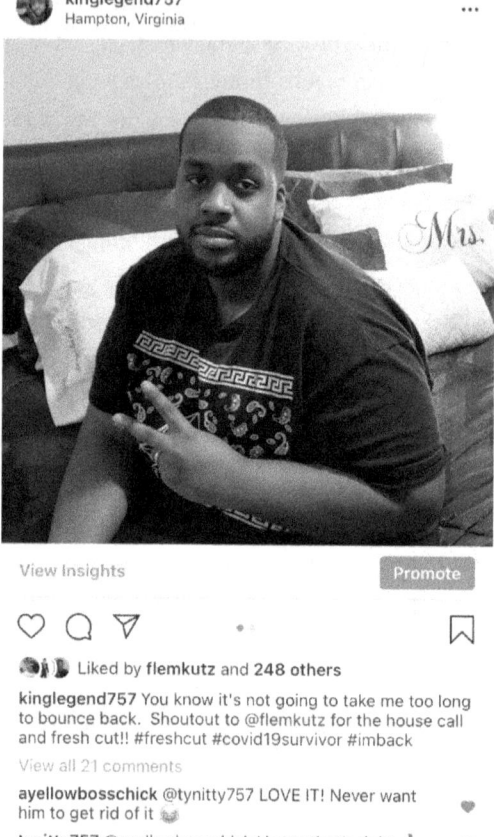

Chapter Eight - Depression

There are many feelings that can cause a person to be depressed. I would not compare my level of depression to someone with a clinical condition. After all, depression is truly a state of mind. The only thing about life that is guaranteed is the fact that it will go on. Even when you are buried six feet deep below the surface, there will be people walking over you above the grass.

You may ask the question, "What is there for you to be sad about?" The answer is more complicated than just one sentence. There was a time during my recovery where I began to feel useless. I was so used to doing things on my own, it became challenging to ask somebody else for help. Something as simple as walking to the kitchen now required a lot of energy, and by the time I made it back to the couch, I would experience fatigue as if I had just run around the house.

The constant pain in my shoulder made it almost impossible to get comfortable in bed or sitting down on the couch. I remember putting icy hot crème on it throughout the day to ease the pain. There were times where I would stay in the house for weeks, only leaving to go to doctor appointments. I remember my first time sitting outside on my front porch and staring at my car parked on the street, this feeling came over me like a dark rain cloud and I just began to beat myself up mentally like my life was over because I could no longer do the things I used to do.

I was upset that I needed help with everything. I have always been the type of person to wear my emotions on my sleeve, not showing any signs of weakness. If I were in pain, you wouldn't know it unless it was really severe. I guess I get that trait from my dad. I have only seen him shed a tear once in my entire life. That was when my grandfather passed.

Even then, he literally only shed one single tear. He has always been strong emotionally as far as not showing emotion. My wife often tries to break me out of that habit and force me to show emotion. There are some days where she knows I'm not in the best of moods and want to be left to myself, but she always tries to figure out whatever it is that is on my mind.

Sometimes I would tell her, but other times I would keep it to myself because I'm a believer in complaining does not solve the problem. I truly don't worry about much because I believe all we can do is our best and accept the results that happen. If things were meant to be, they would be.

It's my faith that makes everything work out at the end and my confidence that God has always got my back. In my moment of weakness, I began to remember who I was as a person and had to tell myself that this was not the end of the road for me. Despite a temporary set back, there was a change in my mindset that would spark an explosive comeback, to inspire others to not give up on life!

I had to remember that drive I had before going to the hospital. I knew I had the fight in me to move forward and keep my head up. I remember telling myself that I would not be defeated. From that point forward, I began to focus on the things I could do and not on the things my body was telling me I couldn't. I began to think about different ways to be creative and spread positivity in the world.

I did some real soul searching deep down and tried to figure out what my purpose was for being here. I know God would not save my life for no reason at all. Whatever my purpose is on this planet, it must be really important for him to intervene with my near-death experience. I have always had people tell me, I have the voice of a radio personality, or that I should look into radio broadcasting.

I always ignored them and continued doing whatever it was I was doing. Things were different now; I had time to really focus on content that I could create. So I focused my energy on creating a podcast. I titled the show using the brand I had already developed through my photography, "King Legend." I remember randomly going live on Instagram with professional gym trainer Kim Reeves. We had a conversation about life, our dreams, and our goals. It was truly great vibes and that's where the idea of King Legend Talks came from. Our conversation was so motivating; it inspired my layout for my new podcast.

Each episode of my show would be me conducting an interview of people who were living their dreams but came from the same living conditions of many families today.

The purpose is to shine a light on people from all walks of life, who also had to struggle with life challenges but eventually made it. Many people have told me how I have a story to tell.

I think it's ironic how I had become interested in learning from theirs, and at the same time provide a message of hope to the audience. The podcast began to do great and people began to give positive feedback. Before I knew it, more and more people wanted to be on the show as my special guest.

My very first official episode of King Legend Talks was my conversation with celebrity producer, "Fat Joe" about the coronavirus. We talked about how health is wealth, and how God saved my life for a reason. That was a conversation that not only motivated me to appreciate the second opportunity I had in life, it also inspired me to promote hope in a world that seemed to be in complete chaos.

2020 had been a crazy year, filled with many downhill crises. The tragic death of Kobe Bryant and his daughter in a helicopter crash, the coronavirus spreading like a bad wildfire across the globe, the impeachment of President Donald Trump, the George Floyd incident that had the entire world rioting, looting, and protesting in the streets for justice, and even murder hornets.

The world had enough negativity to go around for years to come. This podcast was a way for me to focus on the blessings we have in life and provide a light at the end of the tunnel for the people who are still fighting to not give up on their dreams. I encourage people to follow their dreams because I believe God put them there. God makes no mistakes and if you are truly following your dreams, then you are doing the work that he wants you to be doing.

    Our purpose in life was created long before we were born. It's easy to think the idea comes from our mind, but in reality, the creator printed that passion you love on your heart. That is why some people are just so talented in doing the things they love.

My first episode of King Legend Talks was with Celebrity Producer "Fat Joe."

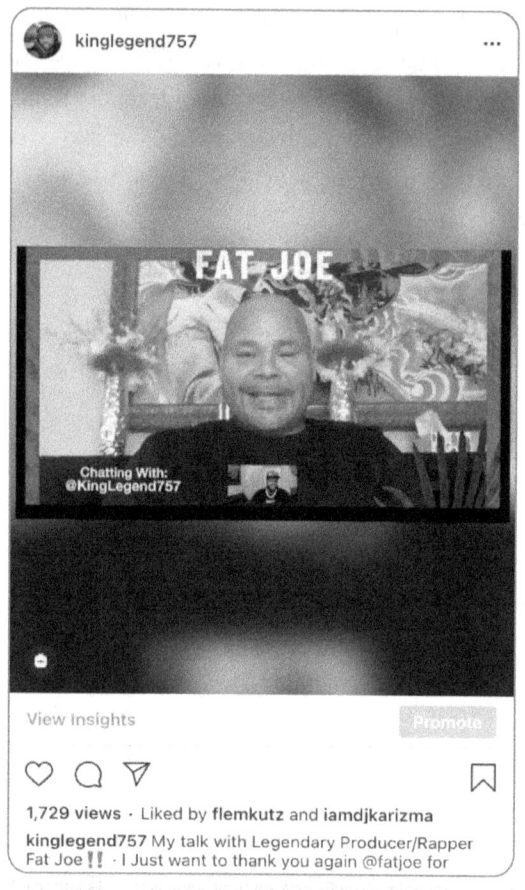

Chapter Nine - Roadblocks

As you can already imagine, the coronavirus has changed my life tremendously. During this part of my recovery, I have had exercised many times with my physical therapist and have progressed to the point of being able to walk down to the end of my street. He had done everything he could do to get my legs to strengthen up. Only a few things were blocking my full recovery.

The fatigue I was experiencing, my feet healing all the way, and my right arm's ability to lift up. After months of waiting, I was finally able to get an MRI done. I went to the hospital with the hope of finding answers, so we could begin treatment and hopefully finally get the ball rolling in the right direction. I never in my life had an MRI done on me, so this was definitely a new experience for me.

I remember them putting me in this big machine that I had very little space in. They clamped this headgear over me so I would keep my neck perfectly still during the scan and then the machine would make this loud drilling sound like at a construction site. I was issued a pair of earbuds to block out the noise. I just remember closing my eyes throughout the entire scan to try and make the time go by faster. If you don't like being in a tight space, and not being able to move freely then you will hate the feeling of getting an MRI done. They also injected contrast in my body, which gave me an internal heat sensation that rushed through my body.

After about 45 minutes of the machine scanning my body, it was finally complete. I remember the feeling of relief as I hoped that maybe after getting the MRI done, they would have answers. To my surprise, the results came back with everything looking normal. Which was good news, but also not so good news because that meant I was back to square one after months of waiting for results.

The next roadblock I would reach in my recovery would be my extreme fatigue. So I had a breathing test set up by my doctor to check my lungs. That test was not as easy as it sounds. Imagine the feeling you get after blowing up hundreds of balloons for a birthday party. The nurse would instruct me to blow as hard as I could and as long as I could over and over again.

The results of that test came back less than normal, but not low enough to trigger any real concern medically speaking. My doctor prescribed me an inhaler for when I feel shortness of breath. I find myself using it maybe once every two weeks or so when I get this weird feeling my blood pressure is high. It makes it hard for me to breathe as I can feel my heart racing.

High blood pressure was one thing that concerned my doctor immediately following my first check-up. I was given medication to fight the blood pressure and for the most part, it is headed in the right direction now. They were even able to decrease my dosage from twice per day, to once a day.

The next roadblock I would face was with the neurologist. He set me up for a nerve test to be conducted. I remember arriving at the hospital in Norfolk, Virginia surprised to see that they had valet parking. When I went inside the hospital and met the doctor who would be doing the test on me, I remember him connecting these stickers like things on my hands.

He would send a small shock to the nerve to see if the correct muscle would respond. He did this on both sides of my body to get an accurate comparison.

When the results from the test came back, it was confirmed a few days later that I had nerve damage in that right arm that controlled the lifting function in my arm. I was happy that the hunt for the issue was finally over, but was not expecting the words that would come out of my doctor's mouth from the follow-up appointment.

He informed me that the nerve damage was most likely caused due to my encounter with Covid-19 and that because of the type of nerve that is affected, it could be permanent damage. He said, there is no way of actually telling if you will ever be able to lift that arm back to normal again.

In other words, it could come back one day but there is no way of actually telling how much of it I would gain back and that there was no cure for my situation, only time would tell. I remember the feeling of sadness that came over me when I heard those words coming from his mouth. This was a tough pill to swallow.

I have faith that things will get better but nobody wants to hear news like that, I don't care how strong you are. I remember my wife trying to be strong for me and not shed a tear, but this is when reality truly set in for me. All this time, I was hoping for treatment of some sort, only to received the news of no cure. After leaving the doctor, my wife drove to the store to get a few items and I remember sitting in the car. For the first time, all the pain and emotions hit me all at once and I actually began to cry. I had been strong all this time and had always kept my head up, but even superman breaks down in the presence of kryptonite. This news was definitely my kryptonite. I ended up calling a close friend on the phone and sharing the news.

Sometimes it's good to have someone not as emotionally attached to the situation to talk to you, so you can see things clearly. We ended up talking about how strong I was as a person and to not forget who was in control of my life. A much-needed pep talks to say the least. Afterward, we ended up joking about movies and our favorite television shows and that positive energy filled my car.

By the time my wife came back to the car from shopping in the store, I had wiped my tears and was ready to move on from the conversation. I just kept telling her that I was ok and that everything would work out. One of the things the doctor recommended I apply for was a long-term disability.

Honestly, I believe that is what made me break down the most. I felt as if, I am too young for that. I was only 26 years old, I felt as if there had to be another way to move on. I don't believe there were too many words exchanged when I got back home that evening between my wife and I.

I believe I put on my headset and zoned out for the most part on the video game for the rest of the evening. Playing video games had become mental therapy for me to block out the noise I was hearing in my head at times.

When my mind needed a break from what was going on in life, I would focus on the game to block out negative thoughts that would try to come inside my head. Thoughts like my arm would never get better, I would be on disability for the rest of my life; or questions like, "Why did this have to happen to me?" I went through major mood swings on days like those. I would be fine and then all of a sudden, I would want to be left alone and unbothered. I began to talk less and seem uninterested in almost everything other than the game.

My wife had a lot on her plate, working vigorously to keep my doctor's appointments organized, and on top of my hospital bills. My wife was with me every day when I first came home until she started going back to her regular job. She works Monday through Friday. She had gotten so used to taking care of me, that she felt uncomfortable the first couple of weeks of me being home by myself.

She would tell me not to try and do too much and if I needed anything, to call her. One day I could feel my blood pressure extremely high and I remember having this shortness of breathe feeling again that morning before she left to go to work. She was so concerned that she sent my brother-in-law to come over to the house and sit with me, to make sure I was doing ok.

One thing I can say about her family is their bond is very close and they support each other with unconditional love. Of course, we all have normal day-to-day family issues that may pop up, but they always come back together eventually. That's one of my favorite things I love about her family. They definitely got our back, regardless of the situation.

I remember when Mother's Day was coming around. I promised myself that I would go visit my mom despite how I felt. I had not seen my mother since being out of the hospital and was determined not to miss the opportunity of spending a moment of that day with her.

My parents are older in age, and I am the youngest born of four brothers and zero sisters. My wife drove me over to my parent's house on mother's day and I saw both my parents and one of my brothers for the first time since coming home. My parents were so happy to see me alive and well. It was definitely a great moment; I even got to take a picture with my dad and mom together in it.

That was a rare thing with my dad. He never did take a lot of pictures with family. He pretty much always stayed to himself when it came to stuff like that. Crazy how life works out, the only person I ever wanted to make proud of on this planet was my pops. Gaining his approval has always been a life long milestone for me.

I guess that's what kept me out of trouble all of these years and always motivated me to do the right thing. I'm proud of you is one thing every son, wants to hear his father say to them. Just like every daughter would love to hear those words from her mother. I have come to realize that it doesn't matter how many roadblocks you encounter in life, as long as you don't let those obstacles in your way defeat you, and end up losing your path to success when en route to your destination.

We must fight the good fight of faith and believe we can come out of any situation victorious with our head held high. My recovery process has been filled with roadblocks, which will eventually be turned into stepping-stones I will walk over with pride and dignity. Nobody ever said the road to recovery would be easy. In fact, it has already been proven to be difficult. Only the strong will survive, I am strong. Like Rocky Balboa said, " It's not hard you can hit, it's how hard you can get hit and keep moving forward. That's how winning is done!" Life can hit hard at times, but God made us strong enough to take the punches.

THIS WAS THE PICTURE I TOOK WITH MY MOM ON MOTHER'S DAY!

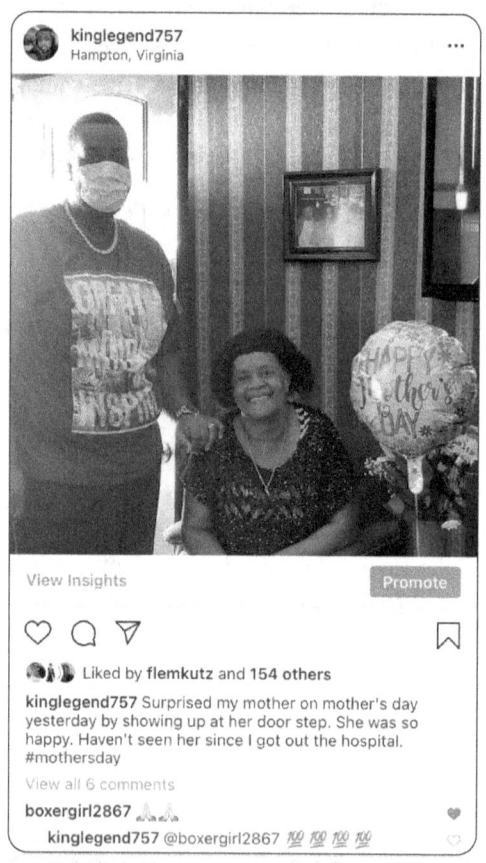

Chapter Ten – Reflection

Sometimes in life, the only way to see progress is to look back on the obstacles you have been through. When you have a lot going on at one time in the moment of things, it's easy to overlook all of the success you have actually achieved. This is the reality of enduring a long journey on any road to recovery. There are times I find myself thinking about why is it taking so long. The constant fatigue, nerve damage, and what seem to be a stop in a pause in my feet healing back to 100%. Then I have to tell myself, death is permanent.

I truly survived life-threatening symptoms; I could have died of double pneumonia alone. So I must take the blessing of life God gave me, and be thankful for every breath I am able to take.

Many people in the same shoes were not so lucky and lost their lives to the virus. I remember looking at the number of deaths rise to the virus and ask myself, "Why did they have to die?" It used to make me feel so weird at times. This virus is so unpredictable; some of the people who died were in better physical shape than me.

To survive something that so many people have died from can have a mental effect on you. It can make you feel a sense of urgency to be more responsible with the life you have left. Tomorrow is not promised. Of course, we hear this all of the time, but surviving death gives it a whole new meaning. A lot of people ask me, "Do you feel any different about life after surviving Covid-19?" As if my relationship with God would be any different now that I dodged a bullet. In all honestly, I don't feel it should change at all. There was nothing he did for me, that I didn't already know he could do. My faith has always been strong, and I have always placed every bit of my confidence in Jesus Christ.

I know some of you reading this may have different faiths or beliefs. I just know my belief in Christ has never let me down before. I have no reason to doubt what I believe in, and that is enough for me to live by. So don't ever get it twisted when I say the doctors saved my life. In truth, it was the calling God gave them to be caretakers. In my opinion, he knew which one of those doctors who would care for me before they were even born.

What if they fulfilled their purpose on this planet by going to school to become the caretakers they are today, just to keep me alive? Living life with purpose is more valuable than any amount of money one can obtain. When you have found your purpose in life and pursue it daily, you are actually doing what God wants you to do. That's why I encourage people to follow their dreams; I believe God put them there.

Looking back on how weak my body actually was when I was in the hospital compared to now, I have come a long way. I really had to learn my motor skills again. Stuff as simple as sitting up in bed, standing on my own two feet, walking to the bathroom, swallowing my food, picking up my own cup to drink water from, and even speaking normally. Nurses would actually have to come to clean me up like a baby that needed his diaper changed. The idea of that happening to me at only 26 years old is unbelievable.

The top three things I would say I really hated about my experience in the hospital are, the ventilator being number one, my hallucinations at number two, and being stuck in the bed not being able to care for myself at number three. I can't express to you enough how God is Great. He has helped me get through the very most this year in 2020. Again, I have to give my utmost respect to the staff at Sentara Hospital who played their part in my recovery.

I am so happy that I had people watching over me who were passionate about their careers. If they had treated me with little intentions of doing what they could to keep me alive, then I would probably not be here right now. I believe all of them gave it their best shot as they do every patient. At the end of the day, only time will tell.

This is the hard part about being a Doctor in the medical field dealing directly with patients. The mental abuse their mind must go through daily, I can only imagine. Trying not to get attached to patients for some doctors is like telling a human, not to be attached to oxygen. That's in human nature to want to live, just like it's on every true caretaker's heart to want to save every life possible.

The reality of not being able to save a life, after making every attempt possible to save it must be hard.

So as long as I live, I will always pray for the outstanding caretakers of the world. That is why it is so important to not make their jobs harder by being so careless of how we treat life. Every human born on this planet has value as long as they are breathing.

Nobody is perfect on this planet, and we have many issues that we need to work on as a species, but one thing that should always be the top priority for everyone is preserving life. Regardless of race, gender, or faith, we need to spread love not hate. We should hate things that threaten human life. If people hated the things that caused destruction, depression, and influenced evil, the world would be a better place. It has to start with each of us as an individual.

Life is more precious than what we give it credit for; just think about how many people had to meet before your parents came into existence to bring you into this world. All it would take is one person in our ancestry to have not met, and your entire existence wouldn't have been possible. So to believe you have no value or purpose on this planet would be an offense not only to the creator but also to all the hard work and timing put in place to get you here on earth.

So if you care about life and want to help preserve it, wear a mask. Even if it only helps decreases your chances of catching the coronavirus by 20%, wouldn't you say it's worth it? Considering how precious life is, and how you only get to live once. It's not going to kill you to wear a mask, but I know what could kill you or others if you refuse to protect yourself as much as possible. This virus has no preference. It works under the Grim Reaper Administration. Their principles are the same: it doesn't care if you're young, old, short, tall, skinny, fat, or muscular. This virus is pure evil and is taking the lives of people daily all over the world. Until we have a cure, we must do all we can to fight this evil, not ignore it and say it does not exist. Look at wearing a mask, washing your hands more frequently, and social distancing as if you are putting on your boxing gloves willing to fight back. We have to start somewhere, and as of right now this is the best we know-how.

Chapter Eleven – What Now?

I always tell people that I wouldn't wish the coronavirus on my worse enemy and that's the truth. It's crazy to me how it can affect everyone differently. It may be fatal for one person, and just a minor cough and loss of taste to the next. Since recovering from my major symptoms and issues such as kidney levels being high and getting my blood pressure back under control, I still am currently fighting the constant fatigue and nerve damage to my arm. We have already discussed the nerve damage, but now I would like to explain the constant fatigue.

One of my doctors decided to get a sleep study conducted on me, because based on what I was feeling; I was showing signs of sleep apnea. I did an at-home study. Basically, they give you this small device to wear on your face while you sleep and it tracks how many times you are breathing while you sleep. Sleeping with the device wasn't too bad; it just took some getting used to. I was instructed to have the program on the device running for at least eight hours and not have any caffeine after 2pm. After the results came back from the study, it was confirmed I have a case of severe sleep apnea.

The sleep study showed that in about every minute I am asleep; there are a total of 30 seconds in between breaths that I stop breathing. If you do the math on that, it will equal up to a total of 30 minutes on every hour that I stop breathing. They also found out that my oxygen levels drop all the way down to about 70% while asleep. This was very disturbing news and they requested that I be put on a CPAP machine immediately.

To be honest, I am not looking forward to wearing this machine to bed every night for the rest of my life, but it's all part of the process of living a healthier life. Before my diagnosis, I had no clue how important it is for your body to get proper rest and oxygen at night. Treating sleep apnea can lower your risk of cancer, reduce depression, and increase energy levels by feeling fully rested after sleeping, and also decrease snoring.

The signs of having sleep apnea are loud snoring, lack of energy, daytime sleepiness, and morning headaches. I was experiencing all of these symptoms after having the coronavirus except morning headaches. Also since recovering from the virus, I have been more aware of my blood pressure and breathing. Sometimes I can feel shortness of breath when I lay down and I have to sit up, just to open the airway in my lungs.

At other times of the day, I can feel if my blood pressure is high and I need to take my medicine. As far as the feeling in my feet, they are sharp pain in three areas at the bottom of my feet that is taking its time healing. The wound care doctor gave me instructions to stay off of my feet as much as possible and to keep them elevated when I am in bed. I explained to him that it is hard to stay off of them because walking around on them as part of my physical therapy. I had to gain that muscle mass back that I lost from not moving at all on the ventilator.

I still am nowhere near as physically active as I was before this crisis, all the sitting on the couch and playing video games create a lazy environment to gain that weight back in. Especially when I find myself always ordering Door Dash. Lately, I haven't been ordering from them as much though. Hopefully, by 2021 I will be able to get back in the gym and get some real workouts going.

Sometimes I think about joining the boxing gym again. I was in the best shape of my life, back when I was boxing. I felt the need to be in shape because it made me a better fighter. Hitting the gym at that time in my life was because; it made me a better athlete. Now I have to hit the gym because it will make me a healthier person and give me the chance to live longer. I think about my health every day since my battle with Covid-19.

To say the least, it made me more consciously aware of the importance of taking care of your health. I remember my conversation with Celebrity rapper Fat Joe when we were discussing Covid-19. He told me a story about the time he was riding a bike on a really hot day in Miami, and how he almost fainted. He said to me, "I'm laying on the grass, looking up trying to catch my breath because my body overheated, it was 100 degrees and I was riding my bike. That's when it really hit me that health is wealth. Everything else means nothing, if we ain't got health, we ain't got nothing."

He also explained how it doesn't matter how rich you are, or how many materialistic things you have, if you don't have health, all of that means nothing because you can't take it with you when you die. Being healthy is much more important to me now than it ever was to me in my life before. People seem to think you can only be addicted to drugs. In reality, addiction is not being able to easily stop doing something that is hurting you, because of the lack of self-control.

You can be addicted to food, gambling, drinking, smoking, video games, and even weight loss. So it can be easy to look at someone who has an addiction to something and say just stop doing that. But in reality, it would be equally hard for all of us to stop anything in life we are addicted to. Words are easier said than done, that's a fact.

I have been saying I am going to get back in the gym like a broken record since I stopped boxing. Working out was never the hard part for me. It was always my diet. I have trained my body to eat until I feel full. Having a set portion size was never my thing. For example, the serving size of a mini bag of Lays Potato Chips is 1 ounce or about 15 chips. That equals 180 calories per serving. So if you're used to eating a normal size bag of chips, you're already almost at your daily calorie intake by just eating one snack. This has always been my struggle with calorie counting.

So I guess you can say if I had an addiction to something it would be food. My diet is very basic, chicken, chicken, and more chicken. Haha, that is not a typo. I eat baked chicken, fried chicken, grilled chicken, and however else people eat chicken. If I took the chicken out of my diet alone, that would eliminate 70% of my bad eating habits. God made chicken taste so good, I had to put it in my book.

I think it's so ironic how everyone thought 2020 was going to be about 20/20 vision and the year of clarity. Now that I think about it, maybe it was. As a country we have exposed things that were going on in the dark, we witnessed the countless amount of deaths to a global pandemic, our government, as we know it has been under constant attack.

The entire nation has been on lockdown and schools have shut down along with large gatherings of any sort. Not just a crisis in the United States of America but all over the world. Nigeria, Africa is almost on the brink of war fighting to end SARS. Negativity has been placed on the big screen for the entire world to see. Is this the clarity the year 2020 has to show us? What can we expect with 2021 just around the corner? I just hope that people decide to wake up and start treating each life as if we are on the verge of extinction. We must preserve the moral values and good behaviors we possess. Treating people with respect, dignity, and honor.

I know there are still good people left in the world because I talk to them daily. I encourage people to hang around others who will motivate you to be a better person. We must build each other up, not tear each other down. Put out a helping hand, not throw a closed fist. We should go back to the basics, if you don't have anything good to say, don't say anything at all.

Social media has changed that mindset of many people in today's society. It's so easy for people to interact with people they do not know and hurt the feelings of people they do not care about. You can be all the way in California and the comments of someone who does not know you all the way in Virginia could ruin your entire day if you let it. We need to stop worrying about things beyond our control and focus on the things that we can. We can control our mind, health, and soul. If each person would focus on growing in a positive way that would ultimately make the world a better place.

So to answer the question at the beginning of this chapter, "What now?" My goal is to bounce back better than I was before. This entire experience with Covid-19 was just a wake-up call to remind me that our days are numbered, tomorrow is not promised and we must not procrastinate on the things we set out to accomplish. If you set a goal, go out and get it done. The last thing you want to do is have regrets as you lay down hoping a doctor can figure out a way to give you more time on this planet. Doctors aren't God, so you better have a good relationship with the man upstairs before you leave and stop taking chances of playing with your life.

Chapter Twelve – Intervention

2020 has shown us how life is like a vapor. It can be here right now and gone in an instant. Nobody could have told me in December 2019 that I would be fighting for my life 3 months later in a hospital. This stuff hits you when you least expect it. Treat people right and show them, love, while they are here. That's when they need it the most. I have been blessed enough to see who actually cared about my life when I was in a crisis, and also who was absent in my time of need. I was also blessed enough to see, who is still checking up on me, and those who are not.

It's not every day you get to witness who will actually show up to your funeral. I thank God every day for the people who still show that they care or were praying for me while I was on the ventilator because I know that they did that willingly from their heart. Having a near-death experience gives you a different perspective on life. It's so weird having a voice in my head that goes off when I feel someone is showing fake love.

To be real, people have always done that but I have always ignored that because it's normal. Just like when people ask you, "How are you doing today?" and then walk off before you can say, "I'm doing fine." Did they really care about how you were doing? Or were they just being polite, so they can say they spoke to you? My biggest fear of this pandemic is that our youth will lose out on human interaction skills. As new technology develops to counter the way of living due to the pandemic social media has already changed the world, as we know it. There are so many people spending their time on mobile devices video chatting and texting. We are moving towards a virtual reality just like in a futuristic sci-fi movie. Television shows now have virtual audiences, sporting events have empty stadiums and everything is going digital.

There is a shortage of coins in the country, and the value of the US Dollar is going down every day. Democracy is at risk, and this pandemic shows no signs of slowing down. All of this stuff is happening right now in our faces and nobody seems to notice. Before we can focus on one issue, it seems another bigger situation takes priority over it. Kids aren't able to play outside as much due to social distancing, and it's for their own safety. The truth is, they are too many issues to address at once. We must put out the fire in our own home before can help our neighbor put out the fire in their kitchen.

I feel like our country needs to focus on unifying the nation. We are more divided now than at any other time I have ever witnessed in my lifetime. At this point in politics, I don't think it matters what is best for people. It seems to only matter who side are you on. A country divided against itself will not stand. We must find a balance before we can move forward and focus on other issues. The left leg is no better than the right leg if together they cannot walk. In politics, that would be the Democratic and Republican parties. They should be able to agree on something, considering the fact the entire nation is involved.

Donald Trump has recently caught Covid-19 after telling people he does not wear a mask everywhere he goes. For most people that may have gone over their heads, but for me, it serves as proof that wearing a mask does help those who believe it or not. According to reports, he has beaten the virus and is clear now. He made a short speech about how he had the virus and how it was nothing. He explained that he got over it because we have some of the best doctors in the world.

He unknowingly, completely dismissed the thousands of people who have lost a loved one to the virus. I say all of this to say this, yes it is true that you can have the virus and be completely fine. You can recover from it with zero complications, but remember that if you are able to experience Covid-19 in that way, you are truly blessed. Count your blessings, because the same virus you may have had and beaten with no sweat, is the same virus that is out here killing people all over the world.

So I would like to take the time to thank the people who wear a mask because they respect the health of others well being. I thank the many first responders who put their health at risk daily to help others and go unnoticed. I thank all of the coronavirus survivors out there willing to raise awareness of the virus despite people protesting in the streets, yelling it's their right to not have to wear a mask.

I thank all of the people willing to listen to the warning signs out there instead of putting themselves and other people at risk of catching the virus. I thank all of the people who don't treat people who have caught the virus any less than people who haven't. Let my story be a message of hope, but at the same time and alarm to remind you this coronavirus is a real thing and should be taken seriously.

We should handle this virus not with fear, but with wisdom and faith that God will make a way when there seems to be no way. God is real. You can count on that! If you made it to the end of this book, please feel free to share it with another. As Denzel Washington would say, "Each one, Teach one."

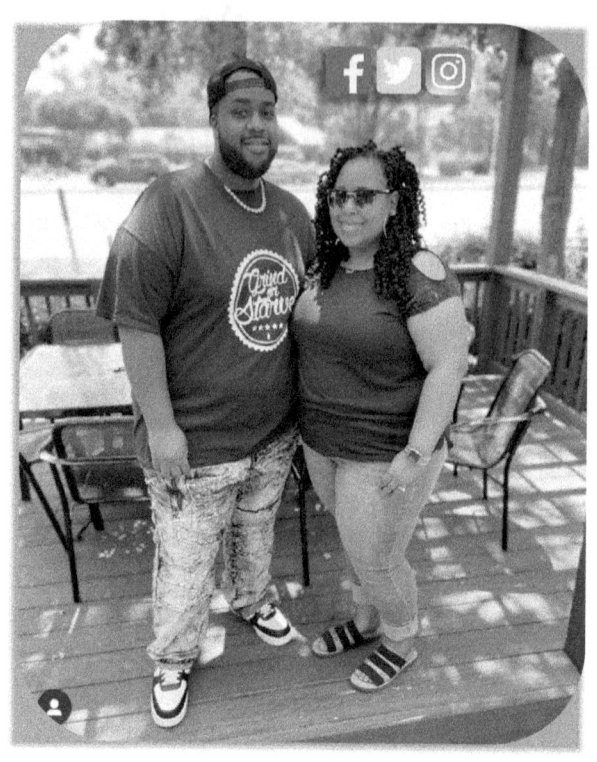

<u>Since we are all living in a digital age where everything is shared on social media, please take a Selfie of you holding this book and share it with a friend on social media. You can tag me in the photo @Kinglegend757 and I will share it to my page as a thankyou for your time and support.</u>

Thankyou for Reading, You have made it to the end of the Book.

Frequently asked Questions...

Did you ever think you would catch Covid-19?

--Honestly, around the time I caught the coronavirus it was the most talked about thing on the news. I was doing my very best to prevent myself from catching it. You could say, I was already social distancing and wearing a mask. Still to this day, I don't know how I caught it.

What advice would you give someone who is feeling symptoms like lost of taste or having a consistent fever?

-- Go to the hospital immediately and get a second opinion, even if you have already gone and were sent home, go again! It could save your life. I went to the hospital two times before catching double pneumonia.

How does it feel to have nerve damage to your right arm? Is there any progress?

-- Having nerve damage to my right arm has definitely been a life changer for me. I have since having it, adapted to what I am capable of doing and am happy for the mobility I still have left in that arm. It has been months and at this time, small progress is being made.

Frequently asked Questions...

Did you experience shortness of breath?
-- I had a hard time breathing at one point while I was experiencing my early symptoms. It felt as if I was in a room with very little oxygen and was very humid.

What is it like knowing you came so close to death and is still here to tell your story?
-- It is definitely a blessing and I live every day happy that God gave me a second chance to live my life. Sometimes I sit outside and just smile at how blessed my life is.

Do you still have fatigue now?
-- Yes, I still feel constant fatigue but I believe it is due to my sleep apnea and that is a current work in progress. CPAP machine is on the way, so only time will tell.

What should you do if you have been in contact with someone who had the virus?
-- You will be fine as long as you don't have any symptoms that follow. To be on the safe side, if possible complete a exercise social distancing and wash your hands frequently.

Frequently asked Questions...

How does Covid-19 spread?
-- It is possible that COVID-19 may spread through the droplets and airborne particles that are formed when a person who has COVID-19 coughs, sneezes, sings, talks, or breathes. There is growing evidence that droplets and airborne particles can remain suspended in the air and be breathed in by others by distances over six feet.

What was the worse part about being on a ventilator?
-- The preparation for getting on the ventilator is the worse part; nobody likes to shove stuff up his or her nose.

What are some things that are common with people after they recover from the virus?
-- Fatigue, low energy, nerve damage to certain body parts and shortness of breath.

How do I stay safe during the Covid-19 Pandemic?

- *Wash your hands often*
- *Avoid close contact with people outside of your home*
- *Cover your nose and mouth with a mask when around others*
- *Minimize contact with those who are sick*
- *Avoid touching your eyes, nose and mouth*
- *Stay home when you are sick*
- *Cover your cough or sneeze with a tissue, then throw the tissue in the trash*
- *Clean and disinfect frequently touched objects and surfaces using a regular household cleaning spray or wipe*
- *If you suspect you may have COVID-19, call ahead before visiting your doctor*

COVID-19 affects different people in different ways. Infected people have had a wide range of symptoms reported – from mild symptoms to severe illness.

Symptoms may appear 2-14 days after exposure to the virus. People with these symptoms may have COVID-19:
- *Fever or chills*
- *Cough*
- *Shortness of breath or difficulty breathing*
- *Fatigue*
- *Muscle or body aches*
- *Headache*
- *New loss of taste or smell*
- *Sore throat*
- *Congestion or runny nose*
- *Nausea or vomiting*
- *Diarrhea*

Look for emergency warning signs for COVID-19. If someone is showing any of these signs, seek emergency medical care immediately:
- *Trouble breathing*
- *Persistent pain or pressure in the chest*
- *New confusion*
- *Inability to wake or stay awake*
- *Bluish lips or face*

www.ingramcontent.com/pod-product-compliance
Lightning Source LLC
Chambersburg PA
CBHW070807220526
45466CB00002B/588